Listening to the Waves

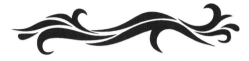

Regan Nicole Brady

Published by

ISBN-13: 978-0-615-43106-2

For more information, visit www.listeningtothewaves.com

This book is dedicated to:

My family,
those who helped to make this book possible, and
everyone who has helped me along the way

Contents

Foreword

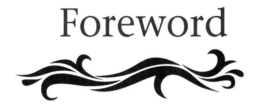

There are certain children a clinician meets along one's shared journey that changes one's life. Regan Nicole Brady would be one example of that unique individual. Although I spread the word that "the sky is the limit" for children who are deaf or hard of hearing—Regan is one who truly epitomizes that mantra! She is a child first—a smiling, pretty, smart, interactive, sweet and truly kind young person—who just so happens to be profoundly deaf. And her future is tremendously fantastic. All because her parents and family, along with a host of experienced professionals who made up a team addressing her testing and management of all her audiologic, amplification, and cochlear implant needs; and most importantly Regan herself, who with perseverance and lots of hard work—believed that she had every possibility and potential to learn to listen and develop spoken language. All these wonderful efforts have resulted in a wonderful person, who listens like a hearing child, has the same (or better) speech skills of any child her age, and the spoken language abilities of a much older youngster. Her contribution with this book which will help other families and children who have hearing loss just adds to how proud I am to say, Regan, you are unbelievable. I am so proud to be your friend!

Donald M. Goldberg, Ph.D.
Co-Director, Hearing Implant Program
Cleveland Clinic, Head and Neck Institute

President, AG Bell Academy of Listening and Spoken Language

Introduction

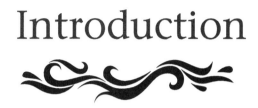

Hi! My name is Regan Nicole Brady. I wrote this book to tell you a little bit about myself and my hearing loss. My family and I came up with the idea of writing a book about myself so that we could share my story with parents of other deaf children, children who are hearing impaired, or just anyone who is interested in learning about a young girl with two cochlear implants. When I was diagnosed with a hearing loss, there were not many resource books that talked about what daily life was like with a hearing impairment. My parents were looking for information on what my life might be like growing up deaf, rather than all the technical stuff out there. I honestly believe myself to be a hearing person, because

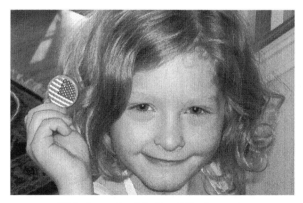

This is me just before Kindergarten with a sticker on my BWP headpiece!

I always wear my implants. The only time that I take my implants off are when I take a bath/shower, swim or when I go to bed. Even then, I don't think of myself as a deaf person, because I grew up hearing with my implants and it seems "normal" for me. I think that the only people that may view me as being deaf are the people on my swim team, because in the water, I cannot wear my implants. I believe that I am really successful with my implants and I want to share my story to hopefully help someone else be successful. I hope that my story will be very useful to you, and I wish you lots of luck on your journey to find the best for yourself or your child!

A bit about myself

First, my name is Regan, pronounced like the former President Ronald Reagan, but spelled with just one 'a'. I wouldn't want you to read this whole book pronouncing my name wrong! Actually, I wasn't named after the former President. My parents had met a family while on vacation in Arizona with a baby named Regan. My mother really liked the name and after 36 hours of labor with me, my dad said she could pick my name!

Birthday: January 6, 1999 (Capricorn)

Age: 11 years old

Grade: Starting 6th grade

Eye color: Blue

Hair color: Strawberry-blond, sometimes curly and sometimes wavy.

Residence: I live in Shaker Heights, Ohio

My First word: "Simba," the name of our cat..

Interests: People- they're very fun and interesting to look at! I like watching people in busy places like malls or in the city.

Fears: I know it sounds silly, but I am afraid of the dark corners of rooms, where Harry Potter characters can jump out and harm you in your sleep! I also dislike small dogs that nip at your heels and bite your feet, and all slimy creatures!

Family members: Sharon (mom), Corey (dad), Ryan (sister who is 7), Toby (our large Golden Retriever), and Simba (our old cat).

Activities: Swimming, soccer, church choir, Crooked River Ensemble, ski club, guitar, tennis, golf, reading, piano, and singing all the time!

Hearing loss: Bilateral severe-profound sensorineural

First Cochlear Implant: 21 months old/Advanced Bionics 1.2 body worn platinum processor (BWP)

Second Cochlear Implant: 7 ½ years old /Advanced Bionics 90K Ear level Harmony processor (BTE)

Pet name for implants: "My Sounds"

Disabilities: Deaf

Abilities: Endless...

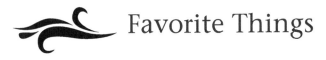 Favorite Things

Foods: Ben and Jerry's oatmeal cookie chunk ice cream, brownies, cookies, and anything at The Chicago Chop House! Almost anything involving butternut squash or pumpkins, like raviolis and soups.

Singers: Taylor Swift, Jason Mraz, Cheryl Crow, John Denver and many more.

Books: Probably *Isabel of the Whales* by Hester Velmans or *Trumpet of the Swan* by E.B. White. It is hard to have a favorite book, because I have read so many! I am currently reading the *Fablehaven* series by Brandon Mull. I enjoy historical fiction, Sci-Fi and fantasy books.

Movie: All 3D movies, *Up,* and *Pirates of the Caribbean*

TV shows: My sister, Ryan, and I like to watch *Ninja Warrior.* This is a game show where the contestants try to race their way through a crazy obstacle/adventure course without falling into the water below. The show is narrated in Japanese and captioned in English. I decided that I like shows that are captioned because I don't miss things. I suppose I should expect to miss a lot of things when announced in Japanese, since I do not speak Japanese! Anyway, I think captioned television shows and movies are helpful to probably everyone. I also like to watch *A Minute to Win It*, which is a show where a contestant is selected to do a completely wacky task in one minute, such as keeping three feathers in the air for 60 seconds using only their breath, or dipping their nose into Vaseline to transport cotton balls from bowls on one side of the stage to the other. This is such a funny show to watch! My favorite cartoons are *Tom and Jerry* and *Sponge-Bob*.

Colors: The rainbow!

Lucky Numbers: 6 and 11

Car: Nissan Cube or Volkswagen Beetle

Places: The Outer Banks in North Carolina, Rawhide in Arizona (an old western town), Chicago, or Miami Beach. I tend to like all of the places that I have been to!

What I Know About My Hearing Loss

I am deaf due to a dysfunction of the hair cells in my inner ear. My deafness is genetic, caused by a problem with a gene called Connexin 26. My family had no idea that I had a hearing loss until I was about 9 months old. It was my father who first thought that something might be wrong with me, although he wasn't sure what was actually wrong. I was a smart baby but something seemed a little off. He said that I never really reacted to them when they came in to my room in the morning until I saw them out of the corner of my eye. My parents began doing little self-tests on me to see if I was hearing okay, but I was a tricky kid and my parents couldn't figure it out on their own. The first place my parents took me to was to my pediatrician. She did not think anything was wrong with me, but said that if my parents were worried, that I should be seen by an ear, nose, and throat doctor.

The ear, nose, and throat doctor could not find anything wrong with me either, but referred us to an audiologist. The next few months were very hard on my parents as they tried to figure out what was going on with me. Sometimes it seemed like I could hear and sometimes it seemed like I could not. One audiologist was convinced that I had something called auditory neuropathy. Of course this led to my parents having to research about that and take me for more tests. We had to go to the doctors our insurance company told us to go to even if they could not do hearing tests, just to be referred to another doctor. My parents said that finally one doctor, a doctor at The Cleveland Clinic, simply asked them if they thought I could hear. "NO!" they both said, so relieved that finally someone wanted to listen to what they thought, instead of just doing things the "medical" way. This doctor then agreed to put tubes in my ears so I could be ready for another type of hearing test. My mom just started crying when the nurse said the appointment for ear tubes would be in a month. They had been going to doctors for three months already trying to figure out what was going on and just wanted answers. The doctor agreed to put my ear tubes in the next week and then I had to have a test called an ABR. The ABR test would see if my brain would react to sound when I was asleep. I was finally diagnosed with a severe – profound bilateral hearing loss when I was 13 months old. My parents were so relieved to finally know what was going on with me. Although the diagnosis was very difficult for them, they finally knew and felt that now they could start to deal with my diagnosis.

The audiologist that did my ABR test and gave the diagnosis to my parents was Dr. Sharon Sandridge of The Cleveland Clinic. Dr. Sandridge told my parents that I would be okay and that I could be taught to listen and speak if that is what they wanted for me. She also recommended that they contact a doctor by the name of Dr. Donald Goldberg who could help with teaching me how to listen and speak. At that time, my parents did not know that Dr. Goldberg was actually Dr. Sandridge's husband (she didn't tell them). I was put into powerful hearing aids within a few weeks and then into digital hearing aids a few months after that. Although I do not remember what it was like to hear for the first time, my parents said that I took off running!

It took some time to track down Dr. Goldberg, but it was worth it! Dr. Sandridge said that she asked Dr. Goldberg to start seeing me because I had strawberry blonde hair like her. I don't know if that is true or not! Dr. Goldberg explained to my parents that I could learn to listen and speak with something called Auditory-Verbal therapy, if that is what they wanted for me.

Therapy

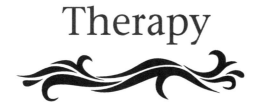

M y parents did a lot of research on communication modes
when they found out that I was deaf. They learned
about sign language and Cued Speech, thought about total
communication and Auditory-Verbal (AV) therapy. My mom attended a few sign language classes and began teaching me made
up signs so that I could communicate with them. I had a sign for 'hi',
'bye', 'fan', 'Simba', 'milk' and 'Teletubbies', one of my favorite
shows. My parents joined a local parent support group called Natural
Communication Inc. and met children who used the Auditory-Verbal
communication mode. Auditory-Verbal is when you use your
hearing to listen and your voice to talk, just like normally hearing
people. AV seemed like the most natural communication method to
my parents. Other communication modes, they thought, would
separate me from other people too much, and not allow me to grow
up as independently as possible. My parents also thought that if

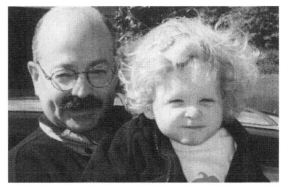

Regan and Dr. Goldberg October 2001.

AV did not work for me, that they could try another way to communicate with me later if they needed to, but that it might be harder for me to do AV later if I had already learned sign language, Cued Speech or something else first because I would not be using my hearing as much.

There had been no other deaf people in my community or my family, with the exception of my great-great grandparents, who passed away a few years ago. I did have the chance to meet my great-great-grandfather. He used sign language, but also talked. He could hear you if you talked really loud. He and my great-great-grandmother had met each other at the Columbus School for the Deaf in Columbus, Ohio. I was the 7th grandchild in my family and no one else had hearing loss. In fact, when my mother was pregnant with me, the nurse said that since hearing loss was so far back in my family history, that they would not test my hearing when I was born. This was before the mandatory newborn hearing screening laws. (The parent group that my parents joined, Natural Communication, Inc. helped to pass the newborn hearing screening laws years later!)

I began Auditory-Verbal therapy with Dr. Goldberg in his basement/office once a week so that I could learn to listen with my hearing aids. There is not much I remember about therapy at Dr. Goldberg's, other than what his basement/therapy room looked like and that he had a dog named Sonoma. We would spend a lot of time in his kitchen baking cookies and I often left with treats. I also remember doing a lot of 'tests' with flipbooks to see what my expressive and receptive language skills were. My mom and dad said that we really just played games—he had a lot of puzzles, board games, and wind up toys to play with. I do remember my experience book. An experience book is like a big scrapbook of my daily experiences. Mine was a big white binder that we would add pages to every few days. My experience book was full of pictures that I drew and photos of places that we went. The idea behind the book was that I would take it to therapy and have to tell Dr. Goldberg what had happened to me. It is fun to look back now at my experience book to see what I remember.

AV therapy was a big part of my life for a long time. Okay, it was my only life! My parents talked and played with me all of the time. We read books together, did puzzles, baked, and sang songs. They pretty much narrated daily life to me in the hopes that some day I would be able to talk back, not back talk! For a period of about a year, my parents also took me to the University of Akron's Audiology and Speech Center for AV therapy. This was a program ran by Dr. Carol

Flexer and Dr. Denise Wray, as well as the students enrolled in the hearing and speech program at The University of Akron. I sometimes also saw Dr. Wray privately. We did all this in addition to seeing Dr. Goldberg because my parents wanted to take advantage of every opportunity they could to help me learn to hear and speak. My parents worked very hard at exposing me to sound, and making sounds meaningful to me. A lot of people think that hearing aids and cochlear implants are like glasses or contacts and once you put them on, you can hear perfectly. When you have a really bad hearing loss like me and never heard before, you have to train your brain to know what sounds are and that sounds have meaning. If you never knew that there was sound, once there is a sound your brain still really doesn't know it is there until it learns to recognize it and link that sound to something meaningful.

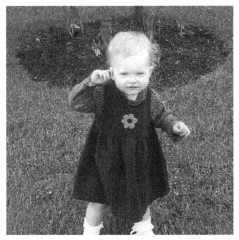

This is me pointing to my ear because
I heard a meaningful sound.

My main therapist was and still is, Dr. Donald Goldberg. I would go to his house and we would always play games or do other forms of practicing together. I would always look forward to my visits, because he would always have something fun planned out for us. Most of my therapy consisted of reading, listening, and playing games—most of all TALKING! I continued AV therapy weekly for a few years, but even Dr. Goldberg will tell you that most of AV therapy is done at home.

There were a lot of other things (and people) that helped me learn to hear and speak. My parents enrolled me in Kindermusik classes when I was very young. I also started playing the piano when

I was four years old. I went to story time at the library and local kids art and dance classes. From the time that I received my first hearing aids my parents played music for me at every nap and bedtime. My mother would sometimes play a CD of bird songs because she thought it would help my brain recognize high-pitched sounds better! My parents also read to me a lot. They said that they tried to read to me at least a hour every night after playing with me all day. I also listened to books on tape at night and in the car. I think this is probably why I was an early reader and love to read! I have many Auditory-Verbal therapists, audiologists, friends and teachers who have all helped me along the way, all contributing to who I am today.

Implants

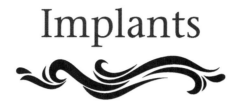

Cochlear implants are what I call "hearing aids with a twist." They are for people who have very little useable hearing. Cochlear implants work differently than hearing aids because they 'go around' the damaged part of the ear to get sound right to the brain. The implant has an internal part and an external part. The internal part of the implant is surgically implanted. It contains an electrode, which is put in position near the auditory nerve. The external part is a processor. My body worn processor (BWP) looks like a big pager and uses a rechargeable battery. The processor converts sounds that come into the implants microphone into a code and that code is sent to the internal device. The internal device sends the coded information to the electrode which stimulates the hearing nerve and that is what my brain perceives as sound. I never like telling people that I have something implanted in my head, but when I do, their reaction is usually, "That's so cool!" You can think of my implant as a way for sound to get to my brain, without having to go through my ears.

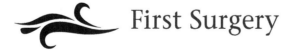 ## First Surgery

I received my first cochlear implant when I was 21 months old. My parents now tell me that deciding on a cochlear implant was the hardest decision that they ever had to make. I was doing very well with my hearing aids. Implanting me was scary. What if it didn't work? My parents attended an AG Bell Convention that year to learn all they could about my hearing loss and especially about cochlear implants. It was really important to them to see how hearing impaired young adults felt about themselves. It was a huge relief to my parents to see other people with cochlear implants perfectly happy! Because my parents and the professionals we were working with felt I would be able to "hear" more with an implant, the decision was made to have the surgery. Dr. Rizer, of the Lippy Group in Warren, Ohio, performed the surgery when I was almost two years old.

I do not remember the activation day of my first implant. My parents said that I just looked up at them as if I were saying: "Wow, this is hearing?!"

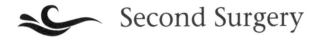 # Second Surgery

My second surgery was the summer after 2nd grade. This again was a very hard decision for my parents. For the longest time, people (surgeons, audiologists) had said to only implant one ear and save the other ear for future technology. It had been 5 years since my first implant and not much had happened in the way of new technology. There had been smaller implants made, like my BTE, but not a cure for hearing loss. My parents felt that if they did not stimulate the nerve on my other side soon that the nerve may die, or at least be harder to stimulate at some point in the future. Also, having two implants would help me hear better and give me a second ear if ever something should happen to my first side.

The second surgery was done by Dr. Peter Weber at The Cleveland Clinic. I remember that I was so nervous that morning, and that I was crying and begging my parents not to take me. I was really scared. I remember I had to wake up so early that morning and that it was raining out. As I waited in my hospital room, I played on my Nintendo DS and tried not to think of what was about to happen. Don came and visited me. He tried to make me feel better about what was going to happen, but it didn't work so well. Friends and family brought presents and the nurses gave me stuffed animals, which I still have today. I had butterflies in my stomach and I was so scared! This time I was aware of what was going to be happening to me as my parents and I talked about the surgery a lot. When it was time for the surgery, my mom came into the operating room with me. The doctors told me to breathe into a mask, and that by the count of ten, I would be asleep. I breathed in that awful smelling gas- it is GROSS and it really gets to your lungs. Lights out! When I woke up, I was being pushed in a bed back to my room. I kind of felt embarrassed because I didn't think I was supposed to be awake yet! Also, I was feeling fine, so I wondered why I was being pushed around in a bed. It was then that I remembered my surgery and I involuntarily moved to touch my head. Yikes! I was all bandaged up with a big foam thing on my head. The bandages were pressing against my ear at a weird angle and it was really hurting now! I was taken back to my room where my parents gave me a sucker, but I couldn't eat it. It was the last thing that I had wanted. I had many visitors including my friend, Riley, who had just had her second implant surgery a few months before. She brought me a WebKinz™ monkey. I slept awhile and when I finally woke up, I realized that I had an IV attached to my wrist. I threw up from the medicine. The band around my head hurt so bad that Dr. Weber had to come in and adjust it. Time had no meaning. It could have been a couple minutes later when they put me into a wheelchair to take me to get into the car, or a couple of hours. Either way, my surgery had gone fine. It took a couple of weeks for me to fully recover and to be able to wash my incision with water. The whole left side of my face was very swollen and for a period of time, I couldn't even see out of my left eye, because it was swollen shut. I rested a lot and read books, and people came to visit. After my head completely healed, it was time to get my second side turned on. I was really excited!

My second processor is called a Harmony. Originally, I was given a processor called an Auria, but it was quickly upgraded to a Harmony, which runs a different speech processing program. The Harmony looks like a large hearing aid and has a rechargeable battery too. I call it my BTE. It was turned on Thursday, June 28th 2006. When it first was turned on, I could not hear words at all. It sounded like a popping noise instead of words. I remembered what everyone had said, that my brain would have to learn what sounds meant since I never heard from this 'ear' before. I thought about what it would hopefully be like some day if it could be as good as my first side. This was the first of many audiology appointments. I left with three different programs to try on my processor, but I really couldn't tell the difference between them. I couldn't even be sure if I was hearing anything out of my 'new' ear or if I was just imagining it. Here are some of my journal entries from that time:

July 5, 2006
The first words I actually hear with my new sound are: baa, cat, push, pea. I practice with flashcards at home. Mostly I still hear popping sounds with a few things that I know are words mixed in. It sounds like each word is popping.

July 9, 2006
Guess what? I heard 18 words with my BTE! Still popping
noises. I try to practice with my BTE.... I am so happy!

July 29, 2006
Problems with my new processor. My microphone broke because
I was bending the ear hook too much so that it would stay on
my ear. I also had to have an electrode turned off.

Here is a chart of what my BWP and BTE consist of:

BWP (Body Worn Processor)	BTE (Behind the Ear)
Magnet inside head	Magnet inside head
Microphone located on headpiece that sits above and behind my ear on my head	Microphone in a discreet location on the earhook (still has the headpiece but without the microphone)
Battery: large rechargeable	Battery: small rechargeable
Processor that I wear in an undershirt	Processor that is worn behind my ear like a hearing aid

**Here are some of the Pro's of doing a second surgery that my
parents considered:**

- I can hear from both directions/sides of my head.
- Hear better!
- Not so dependent on one side- if one implant breaks, we will have the other one!

At night, I take my implants off right before I get into bed. I am supposed to put them in the Dry and Store, but I usually put them on my dresser instead. The reason that I take them off at night is pretty obvious: I take them off so that the processor can rest, and because there is absolutely nothing to hear at night, except for a possible smoke alarm. That leads me to tell you that my dad had a special smoke alarm installed in my room. It has a very bright light and is VERY loud.

I am not a morning person. My parents become very frustrated trying to wake me up in the morning. Every time they come in to wake me up, I fall back asleep again. My sister hears them telling her to get up, but I don't hear anything. My mom ended up buying me a bed shaker alarm clock that shakes my bed really hard. You can put the shaker under your pillow or mattress or whatever works for you and it will shake the whole bed in the morning. They said that I am 'on my own now' but they still help me.

Because my headpieces are only attached to my head by a magnet, they fall off pretty often. They don't just fall off whenever, it's usually when I bump the cord, when I'm changing my clothes or when I'm in gym class. I become frustrated when my cord gets tangled in my usually knotty hair. I'm also frustrated when I'm at school and my implant falls off. I am aware that people might be looking at me, and the fact that I am maybe missing something someone is saying. During these incidents, I usually watch people's lips to see if they are maybe trying to say something to me. Speaking of looking at lips, lip-reading is a skill that I have involuntarily developed over the years. This is VERY useful when swimming with friends, or in noisy places. My parents do not encourage this habit, although I find it useful sometimes, and my friends love to see me do it! I have learned that when people are talking normally, it is easier to lip-read them than when they are talking slowly, "mouthing the words" or trying to exaggerate their words.

There is only one thing that is hard for me to hear, and that is whispers. Whenever someone is trying to whisper something to me, I always end up asking them to a private spot where they can talk to me quietly, instead of whispering. My implants have a volume control and a sensitivity control but I usually do not change them. If I ever do not want to hear, I just take my headpiece or BTE off. Don't get me wrong, I wear my implants ALL the time, but I like to take them off when I am trying to concentrate on something very hard, or sometimes when reading a book. I also take them off when I swim or shower or if I ever go down a plastic slide, to avoid the static electricity. I don't usually go on plastic slides anymore, for whatever reason.

The speech of a deaf person is perhaps the most noticeable effect of their hearing disability. Because their hearing may not be as good as those who don't have a hearing loss, their speech may sound normal to them but not to us. Everyone I meet (that knows that I have implants) always notes my good, clear speech. Further proof to myself of my normal voice is my participation in my church choir and school musicals. I do believe that I hear just as everyone else does. I do think about this a lot: What if two friends were listening to a third friend talking, but one of the listeners interprets it as a different voice, perhaps like a "robot" sound. Meanwhile, the other listener is interpreting it in a different way. What if everyone is hearing things differently than others, but we are unaware? It is easier to understand with colors: What if Sally's "red" is actually Sue's "purple", while this is Sadie's "orange"? The other colors would be different too, because colors are sort of in ratio, like the color wheel. I know that this is very confusing but it is interesting to think about on a rainy day!

It is hard to describe what it is like when my implants are off. Without my sound everything is different, but not in a way that isolates me from the world. It's as if you have a picture in your mind and then it was 'dimmed' as if a screen door closed in front of it. It's impossible for hearing people to imagine what it is like to be deaf. You suddenly become more aware of movement and vibrations and use your other senses more. It is, like I said, very hard to explain. My point is that I am very lucky to have implants and I love to hear!

School

My parents felt that it is important to write about how I ended up where I am educationally. When I was first diagnosed with a hearing loss, my parents thought that I would never be able to be speak or hear their voices. Once I was in hearing aids, they knew that I could go to a regular school and live a normal life. When I was 18 months old, my parents enrolled me in a preschool for a few hours a day, a few days a week. My mom did this for a few reasons—one was to give her a break from talking to me all day long. The other reason was so that I would learn to listen to other people and other peoples' voices, not just my parents. The preschool was small, it only had 8 kids in it and I was the only one with hearing aids. After I 'graduated' that preschool, my parents looked around for the next school to put me in. They wanted to keep putting me in more challenging environments. The next preschool was a little larger and had carpeted floors. My teacher used a speaker system so that I could hear her voice better. After some time in this preschool, I moved on to another that was again a little more challenging for me. I went to five preschools all before I was five years old! I think this was actually a good idea because my parents would always try to put me in a situation that was just a little bit difficult for me so that I wouldn't fail, but where I would have to work to be successful. Each classroom was a little bigger than the previous one with more students and more challenging for me academically so that I would be ready for Kindergarten.

 # IEP

When you are school aged and have a disability, you can go to your local school district and see what services they may have to help you in school. The school is supposed to create something called an Individualized Education Plan to help students with disabilities learn in school. My parents went through the IEP process in our town (Avon, Ohio at the time) but it did not go so well. Because I was the only deaf kid in my community, my school district did not have appropriate services for me. They offered to have me go to school at the county school for disabilities and to work with a speech therapist. Because I had been through years of AV therapy, my parents were sure that I should go to a regular school and that I should have good speech role models. Also, I should have an AV therapist, not a speech therapist. Dr. Goldberg and Dr. Wray visited the programs the school district wanted me to attend and said that they would not be good for me. The school district and my parents disagreed on other things too. My parents felt that the school district should be responsible for the programming of my cochlear implant because if my implant did not work right, I would not hear well and would not benefit from my education. My parents had to go to court against the school district, something called due process. We had many important people that supported us such as Dr. Goldberg, Dr. Wray and lawyers from AG Bell. Guess what? My parents won! This was a huge deal not just for my family, but for families everywhere who were trying to get appropriate services for their children. The hearing officer ruled in our favor saying that programming a cochlear implant was a related service and that the school district was responsible for paying for that. Since the school district did not have these services, they had to reimburse my parents for taking me to my usual audiologist for programming. It was all a matter of principal.

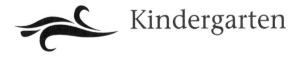 # Kindergarten

My parents rejected placement in the county's disabilities program and placed me instead in Kindergarten at a private school, Lake Ridge Academy. They liked LRA because it had small classes and carpeted rooms, which is good when you have a hearing loss. I went to LRA for my kindergarten year, and my teacher was Ms. Dillon. She was a very nice teacher who allowed me to do harder things than the rest of the class, like read chapter books when everyone else was learning how to read. I used a surround sound in my classroom. The system was called a Radium. It was a tall speaker that sat on the floor of the room. My teacher would wear a headset with a microphone and her voice would transmit to the speaker so that I (and everyone else) could hear better. This worked out well for me hearing-wise. My parents decided that while LRA was a good school, they were not willing to make too many exceptions for me academically—I was ahead of the class in math and reading and my parents wanted to keep me challenged. I really think that because of all of the AV therapy I did, it helped me to become a good student. We switched schools after kindergarten.

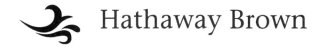 # Hathaway Brown

I started Hathaway Brown School in first grade. HB is a private girls school that has been great for me. When I was in second grade, we moved to Shaker Heights to be closer to HB. All of my teachers used my surround sound in the classroom up until fourth grade. We also had systems for music class, art and Spanish, since these were in different rooms. Fourth grade was my hardest year because of all of the homework! I also started a competitive swim team that year so that took up a lot of my time. Fourth grade was also fun because we took a great trip to Pleasant Hill Kentucky to learn about the Shakers, the settlers of my hometown, Shaker Heights.

I am now in middle school at HB. This year was a big transition year for me. There are many changes in middle school such as changing classrooms and different teachers. In middle school, the day is divided into seven classes, or periods, of the same length. Everyone has their own lockers and an individual schedule which makes you feel so mature! The year is divided into three trimesters, instead of two semesters. Also, we have a lettered schedule, with a certain schedule for each day. There are many new students and the 'old' students are changing. There are new haircuts, glasses, braces, physical body changes, and the attitudes are changing even more. BFF's get into fights, people all rush to buy the same shoes, and so on. Especially in fifth grade, cell phones, ear piercing and Gmail is all the rage! My parents recently bought me a cell phone. I love it because texting is so quick and easy!

I started using a personal FM system this year. It consists of a microphone that the teacher wears and a receiver that I wear plugged into my BWP. The microphone picks up the voice of my teacher and transmits her voice directly to me so that I hear her voice louder than the surrounding sounds. It is very nice because I can control the volume and the teachers voice is only amplified to me. I was nervous to try the FM at first because I thought that it was too direct and that I would only be able to hear the teacher and nothing else. However, when I tried it at the end of my fourth grade year I really LOVED it because it enabled me to hear the teacher as loud as I wanted to even when everyone else was being noisy! I thought this would be a huge advantage for me.

All of my teachers are very nice, and almost all of my teachers use my FM. I do not use it in library, art or gym class. I have never really officially told my classmates about my implants. My teachers know about them because we always meet with them before school starts to discuss my needs, which is basically just using my FM system. My classmates just kind of find out about my implants along the way. When people have noticed my implants, they have said things like:

- 50% say "What's that thing on your ear?"
- 25% say "Is that a hearing aid?" (Pointing either to their ear or my ear)
- 20% say "What's that?" (Pointing to my ear)
- 5% say "What's this?" (Pointing or poking at my BWP)

Can you tell that I like math?

I usually respond by saying that I have a hearing aid, because I think that that is easier for people to understand rather than explaining that I have cochlear implants. Overall, the conversation is not very embarrassing for either of us.

Here are some conversations I remember having about my implants:

With new kids I met at summer camp

Tess: "Do you have a hearing aid or something?"
Me: "Yeah, I'm deaf."
Tess: "Mmm, it must be a really good hearing aid!"

Tess to Erin: "Did you hear Regan is deaf?"
Erin: "Ooh, I feel so bad for you!"
Me: "Don't worry, I'm fine!

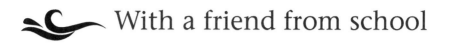

With a friend from school

Leah (who already knows about my implants more than most
people, due to a sleepover at a water park): "Regan, do you
know why there is a carpet under us, but not in the rest of the
classroom?" (We were sitting next to each other in math class
over a tan rug, much like an island. The rug was placed there to
eliminate echoing in the room so that I could hear better).

Me: (Nod) "I'll tell you later."
Leah: "Is it about your…" Leahs words trailed off
Me: "Mmhm."
Leah: "Cool."

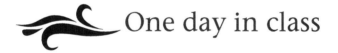

One day in class

Heather, speaking to a teacher: "Why do you wear that thing?"
(pointing to the FM transmitter on my teacher)
Teacher: "Well, I think Regan might want to answer that."
Me: "It's something that helps me hear better in class so I don't
miss anything that the teacher says. It just helps me."
Heather: (Nod, looking embarrassed)

The next day at recess, I told Heather about my sound and we
became closer friends through it. On the way back to the building,
she told me that she would vote for me for student council, because
she thought that I would be the best class representative!

Advice

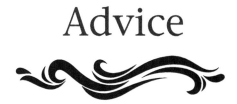

I know how important advice can be when the person giving it has been through the thing that they are giving advice about. That sounds confusing but it is surprisingly simple! You would trust a 5th grader giving advice about 4th grade more than you would trust a 3rd grader giving advice about 4th grade. For those who are still confused, let me explain. A 5th grader has been through 4th grade and the 3rd grader hasn't! That is why I am devoting this section to you-know-what.

Advice for someone who finds out that his /her child is hearing impaired:
1) Believe that everything happens for a reason, although that reason may not be clear.
2) See an audiologist or other professional as soon as possible.
3) Don't feel sad for too long, your baby needs you.
4) Don't blame yourself!
5) Learn about successful hearing impaired people.
6) Get implants or hearing aids for your child to maximize their hearing and learn about all of the communication modes.
7) Don't lose hope!
8) Get a pet. It can help your child (my cat helps me still now with my feelings and is a great pet to have).
9) Find other parents for support.
10) Help your child start a diary. I look back now and wish that I had written one when I was younger.

Advice for People With BWP's and BTE's
1) Wear your BWP in a pocket that is sewn onto an undershirt. I have been wearing my BWP this way since I was 2! Other

people have pockets sewn into clothes, but I like wearing the pocket sewn into an undershirt because it feels like my processor is more secure.

2) Some people like to decorate their implant headpiece or BTE with colorful stickers. This is fine if you don't mind being noticed! One time I was wearing a sticker of a purple butterfly on my headpiece. I was in kindergarten, and someone said that I had something in my hair and they tried to get it out. They accidentally knocked my headpiece off!

3) Do not wear very tight dresses or shirts with a BWP because it will cause a noticeable lump under your clothes. A loose sweater hides the BWP well.

4) Make sure that if you have a BTE, it doesn't fall off when you are playing sports or moving quickly. I use a headband to help hold things in place. If I know I am going to be running around a lot like in a soccer game, I leave my BTE at home. I can just imagine it falling off and being trampled.

5) If you are talking on a phone, it helps you to hear the other person better if you cup your hand around your microphone and the telephones ear piece at the same time to eliminate any background noise.

6) If you swim, a fanny pack is helpful to carry your BWP in when you are on the pool deck. I have also found some nice camera cases that work well. Keeping the implant in a case keeps it from slipping out of your hands and keeps it dry.

7) If people ask you about your cochlear implant or hearing loss, act like it is no big deal and don't be embarrassed. What is there to be embarrassed about? Don't let your deafness define you, you define your deafness!!

8) My body-worn processor has a light that blinks green when sound is picked up by the microphone. In a movie theater or a dark place, it helps to wear dark clothing to block out the blinking light. I once wore a white tee shirt to a movie and lit up the theatre the whole time! (It really wasn't that bright).

9) Always be aware if someone is talking to you, especially in a noisy environment. My parents remind me of this all the time.

10) Ask your audiologist to create a 'noise' program for you to use in noisy places, like restaurants, cafeterias, etc. This shortens the implant's range of sound so that your implant only picks up sounds nearer to you and you can hear better when there is a lot of noise around you. I have a 'noise' program that I sometimes use. It is very helpful.

Heroes and role models

These are some people that I want to be like for the qualities that they possess. These wonderful people are really strong, kind, and determined.

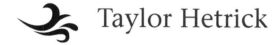 ## Taylor Hetrick

Taylor is a swimmer on my swim team. She is 17 and is blind. I met Taylor at the pool one day as she had just finished a practice. Taylor's mom and sister help her swim by acting as tappers for her. As a tapper, they use long poles with a soft end to tap her on the head when she is getting close to the end of the pool. Taylor then knows to take a few more strokes and then do a flip turn so she will not hit the wall. Taylor and I are the only kids on the team with a disability as far as I know. This past April, Taylor swam in the Paralympics in San Antonio, Texas. Taylor swam 12 events and had 11 best times! Taylor holds American Paralympic records in 50 yard breaststroke, 50 backstroke, 1000 freestyle, 400 IM and 200 butterfly. She also has a long course record in the 400 IM and was invited to represent the US Paralymic team in Greece where she won six gold medals!!!! I am so proud of her!

Seeing someone who works so hard to achieve what she dreams for and doesn't let her disability stop her was really motivational for me. I think it is much easier to be a deaf swimmer than a blind swimmer. I hope that this story of a girl who works hard to reach her goals will encourage you to keep on trying, even if you feel that you can't do it. Taylor really inspires me!

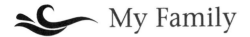 # My Family

My family is my biggest role model, each person in a different way. I look up to my mom because she is so nice, caring, and loving. Although I know that I will never be as efficient as my mother, I will always try to be as time-managed and well planned as her. My father is my role model because he is so funny and easygoing with everyone. I don't want to act fake in front of people, so that they will like me. I want to be myself. Daddy reminds me of that, with his go-with-the-flow manner, which leads me to trying not to be a control freak who wants to always know what is going on! I admire my sister because she is very compassionate (when she wants to be), and has an interesting sense of humor. I want to be as compassionate as her all of the time, and I want to be as funny. My cat reminds me that I always need to get enough sleep and to have faith in God. My dog reminds me to always be happy and optimistic. Most of all I respect myself, and who I am, because that is the most important person to have as a role model. **You are your own hero!**

Some traits that I look for in a role model: Funny; kind to everyone; has lots of friends, but not exclusive; athletic; smart; leader; easygoing; friendly.

Short Stories

Here are some everyday snippets from my life, including experiences, obstacles, and happy moments, just to help you to better understand me...

The AG Bell Convention this summer:

I am very excited to go to the AG Bell convention this summer in Orlando. I am excited for the convention, because this will be my first convention that I will be old enough to remember. I was a baby when we attended the convention in Philadelphia and I don't remember anything except for making paper fans in the kids' program. I am excited to meet other kids my age with implants and I will hopefully be showcasing this book! I am SO happy that the convention is in Orlando because we are planning to visit the Harry Potter exhibit at Universal Studios. I am a big Harry Potter fan! I remember our last visit to Universal in 2006 or 2007 where we saw the signs that the exhibit would open in 2010! I recall thinking that I would never be able to wait that long!

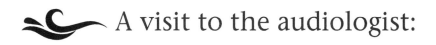 A visit to the audiologist:

I went downtown yesterday for an audiology appointment. There was a new student working with my audiologist, which made me nervous. I have become used to my audiologist and the things we do at our appointments. The student had a voice that was a bit unusual to me. Okay, she had a very heavy accent. First, I had to go into the soundproof booth. Things were fine in the beginning as I was able to repeat the sentences the student said with only my first implant easily. I then became very scared because I had no idea how I could repeat sentences with my BTE. It is still so much easier for me to hear with my original side. When the sentences came, I almost started crying. I knew that she was talking and I could tell the number of syllables in the words, I just didn't know what she was saying. I told her that, but she just kept on going, which I thought was inconsiderate. Then I had to do a test where I had to press a button if/when I heard a sound. It was kind of hard with my left side to know what I was actually hearing and what was my imagination! After that was over, I did more testing to determine the quietest sound I could hear and the loudest most comfortable sound I could listen to. I had to use a chart and point to a number that described how loud the sound was- it was VERY hard to tell the differences between the levels. It gave me a headache after awhile. In the end, after I was given a new program, we did a test called the Ling sounds. When the student with the unfamiliar accent tested the Ling sounds, I couldn't really tell what she was saying. Then my dad did it and I got almost all of them right. I am more used to my dad's voice, which helped me. That was a very long appointment, a good two hours or so.

When I first got my BTE, I was going to the audiologist a lot. My microphone broke a few times because, I found out, I was bending the ear hook too much to try to get it to stay on my ear. I also had some problems with one electrode channel, which I had to have turned off.

I usually only go to the audiologist twice a year now. I try to go right before school starts and then over spring break. When I was younger, I went to the audiologist ALL THE TIME! Since I was little and not really able to tell my parents what I could hear, getting an audiogram was a way for everyone to know what I was capable of hearing. It was important that I was hearing as well as I could with my implant since we were working so hard at getting me to listen and speak. Getting an audiogram before having my implant reprogrammed was important too, so the audiologist could see where changes needed to be made.

I remember when I was in hearing aids that I LOVED to have new earmolds made. It was fun to watch the audiologist mix the material and fill the big syringe with it. I liked the feeling of the mold material in my ear and the audiologist would sometimes give me a piece of the material to play with. I also remember a big poster in the room of all of the earmold colors you could get. One time, at home, my mom had to pull green play dough out of my ear because I was pretending to make my own earmold! Then we had to go to the ENT so they could check that all the play dough was out before I could start using my hearing aid again (he found some).

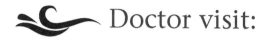 Doctor visit:

 I went downtown on Thursday of last week to have an EKG test and to have my heart checked. I have been having chest pains for awhile. After a few months of chest pain you start to get a little concerned. My pediatrician said that I was just having some muscle pain, but it kept happening every once in awhile and it worried us. My mom scheduled the appointment with my friends' mom, who is a pediatric cardiologist. I was really upset at my mom because I didn't want to have a doctor's appointment with someone that I knew. First I went to have the EKG done. An EKG is a test where the nurse attaches little sticky pads all over your chest, and connects little wires to them. The wires are connected to a machine which reads the electrical impulses in your heart. My EKG was fine. I then went to see my friend's mother. When she went to examine me, she saw my implant in the pocket of my sports bra and asked me what it was. When I told her that it was my cochlear implant, she said that she had forgotten all about that. She said she thought it was a heart monitor! How awesome, thought my mother, that people cannot even tell that I am deaf. My speech is great and I am independent! Whoo- hoo!

 While downtown, my mother had also arranged for me to take part in a FDA study about children and implants. The study is called The ASK CHILDREN STUDY, which stands for Assess Specific Kinds of Children Challenges for Neurological Devices Study. The purpose, from what the study says, is to 'collect information related to neurological devices for children to help identify safety, effectiveness, adverse events and human factors associated with such devices'. The study is supposed to help the FDA understand more about medical devices and make them better for children and adolescents. There are only 110 kids enrolled in the study. Actually the study was just a questionnaire that I had to take home and answer about how I felt about my devices/implants. I probably shouldn't tell you about the questions, but I can tell you that I felt really out of place taking the test because most of the questions did not pertain to me. It asked things like 'do you tie your own shoes?' Not sure how that will help kids with implants! Anyway, I filled out the questionnaire at home and mailed it back. I am supposed to receive a $25 gift card and a tee shirt for completing the study, which I haven't yet! Update: They just came today!

ᴥ Airport Security:

No one likes airport security. Here is how I deal with it. My mom will inform the security officer that I have a medical device that will cause the metal detector to alarm when I walk through. Once we have dumped all of our belongings into the gray plastic bins, we proceed to the metal detector. My mom walks through first and I go next. It seems as if they never really listen to what we have told them, and they act surprised when I set off the metal detector. I carry a card from Advanced Bionics that explains my cochlear implants, but they never look at it.

Then they take me aside to do a wand check, where they wave their metal detecting wand over me to see what is causing the system to alarm. After that, they have to pat me down. More recently they have asked me to touch my processor with my own hands, and then they wiped my hands with a certain type of paper to check for explosives. I felt very aggravated, mad and embarrassed that they did this to me. My mom had tried to show them the card that explained that I had a medical device, but they wouldn't even look at it! They tried to make a really big deal out of checking me over and acted all "cool" as they checked me. I always hate going through security at airports. The metal detector does not harm my implants; it is just annoying to have to endure the wrath of very tight airport security.

When I travel, I always take my battery chargers, a bunch of batteries, and usually my Dry and Store with me. I always pack these things in my carry on bag so they will not get lost!

A very lucky day at camp:

Last summer, I attended a basketball and volleyball camp at my school for one week. It was a fun camp, but one day in particular was awesome! Here is what happened:

1) I won the craziest socks contest in basketball and volleyball camp (luckily the contests were the same day!)

2) In basketball camp, all of the girls with birthdays in January pulled names out of a hat to see who would win a prize. I picked my own name out of about 35 kids and won a cool basketball hoop!

3) My molar fell out (it was still a baby tooth).

4) I won two awards in volleyball camp. One for the best attitude in the whole camp, and one for best listener! AV has trained me well!

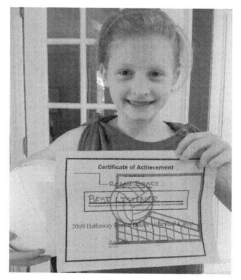

My best listener award!

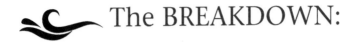

The BREAKDOWN:

On December 1, 2009, my sound (right side) broke down for 30 minutes or so. I took notes when it happened in case I needed to give them to the audiologist. At the time I did not know what was going on and thought maybe it was an internal failure. Here is what happened:

I was at swim practice and dropped my BWP on the pool deck by accident. I didn't think anything of it and went on with practice. After practice, I went into the locker room to change and put my implants back on. Something was wrong with my right implant—it wasn't working right at all. Everything sounded really quiet. I was scared that when I dropped my processor onto the pool deck, it had broken. I tried to change the battery but it didn't help. It seemed as though what I was hearing seemed a bit like my second program, which is my restaurant/noise program. There was a buzzing in the background and everything was so **quiet**. I could only hear loud noises. To make things worse, I was driving home with another family, who didn't know much about my implants so I felt really uncomfortable the whole way home. I just sat there worrying the whole time. At home, we tried different batteries and even an extra processor that I have, but nothing helped. This was a really scary time. Randomly, a bit later, things started working well again. At first things sounded a little echo-like, and then better. Overall, it was a really frightening experience, especially because I had my standardized testing at school the next day and you can't miss that! I believe that it was a signal from God to practice more with my BTE. My parents are always saying that there may be a time when one of my implants might fail and I will need to use the other. I should really practice more with my BTE so that I can hear better with that ear. When I asked the audiologist about it, she said that perhaps it was the humidity of the pool that had affected my headpiece or microphone.

A sleepover experience:

Last night I slept over my best friend, Erin's, house. I was surprised to see as I arrived at her house mid-afternoon, 2 Nerf guns pointed at me! Her two brothers, Jack and William, were aiming them at me! Once the boys decided I was friendly and they would let me by, I ran to see Erin. We spent an hour just talking and catching up on things, and then it was time to get ready for Erin's swim practice. Erin swims for her country club team and invited me to her practice. I figured it would be pretty fun, as I love to swim. I knew that Erin would help me figure out what was going on. Erin was the first girl that I met when coming to Hathaway Brown in first grade. She knew all about my implants and we've had a few sleepovers together, but never a swim practice with other kids and a coach that I did not know! There were lots of kids at the practice that day (Erin said about 40). Erin introduced me to the coach, who seemed pretty nice. It was an EASY practice, seeing that we swam 25's and 50's the whole time! Erin and I developed a system so I would know what we were doing, either she would go first so I would see what to do, or she would tell me, (I would lip read) and then I would pass her towards the middle of the lane so I could keep swimming without running into her. I received compliments on my swimming abilities from the coaches, seeing that I was pretty much the fastest one there! After we swam, we dressed for dinner, which we would have at the country club. Dinner was good, but the brownie sundae was even better! It consisted of a warm brownie, a large scoop of vanilla ice cream covered with warm caramel sauce and all topped off with whipped cream and a cherry. After dinner, we headed back to Erin's house where we played a bit more in her room before going to bed. Erin's bedroom has a wall of windows. I mean a real wall of windows- from floor to ceiling and one end of the room to the other. We slept that night in Erin's room next to the wall of windows, during a horrible thunderstorm. I don't know if I had a nightmare or if it was the lightening that woke me up, but I remember sitting up screaming and Erin's mom running to tuck me in again. I wasn't sure how loud I had screamed because my implants were off, but I was *soooo* embarrassed!

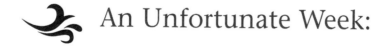 An Unfortunate Week:

One day last week, my battery (to my BWP) went out during my second class of the day. I was surprised this happened since I change into a newly charged battery each morning. Usually, I keep a spare battery in my locker, one in my book bag and one in my coat pocket. I was really panicky and nervous, thinking for some reason I would not have a spare. My teacher was in the middle of demonstrating something, so I had to wait to ask her if I could be excused from class. Although I couldn't hear much with only my BTE, it was obvious that she had said yes. At the beginning of the year we explained to my teachers that I may have an 'emergency' such as this in class. I ran down the hall to my locker, checked my coat, and was relieved to find a battery. I was hoping it was a good one! I put it into the shallow pocket of my pants and ran to the bathroom. When I was almost there, I felt my foot kick something, I looked down to see that my battery, which had fallen out of my pants pocket, was sailing toward the edge of the two-story balcony. *OH NO!!* Please don't let this happen! I then remembered the inch high safety guard underneath the railing, and hoped that it would stop my flying battery. I cautiously peered under the safety guard, afraid of what I might not see. *OH NO!!* It wasn't there!!! *OH NO!!* I glanced over the railing and I saw my battery lying vulnerably on the stairs. I was so glad at this point that it was in the middle of classes and no one was around to see! I quickly checked around to see if a teacher had seen the incident—it was against the rules to drop anything over the balcony! Luckily not! I ran down the stairs, got my battery, HELD IT TIGHTLY, and ran into the bathroom, trembling, where I discovered that... it was a good battery. THANK GOODNESS!

MORE PROBLEMS... I was in the middle of English class, which was my first class that day, and my FM system wasn't working. Aye aye aye ya! (or however you spell that). Another malfunction this week! Anyway, I tried checking what I could, but the FM wasn't working. I knew that the part the teacher was using was on and the battery was good because I recharge it every night. What could be the problem? I had no idea! When I tried to disconnect the FM receiver from my processor, I felt the cable of the FM fall apart. *OH NO!* Not again! This had happened to me in the past. I was a bit relieved that it was only two days away from spring vacation, during which, I could have the FM fixed, but annoyed again that this had happened. For those two days, I was fine without my FM, and I ended up being able to get to my classes faster because I didn't need to wait for the ever busy teachers to give the transmitter back to me at the end of class.

❧ A swim meet:

Sweating in the hot, humid, chlorine-smelling bleachers. Listening to "Beep... Take your marks." Watching the splashes and the 200 IM's. Eating my fruit rollups®, and cheering my friends on.

Where am I? At a typical swim meet! Oh, and one more thing, its 7:30 a.m. Now that I'd just aged up to the 11-12 year old age bracket, I swim in the afternoon sessions at swim meets. However, today, my mom didn't realize that, so here we were, on event 3 out of 20. I was sweating like crazy. "I need to get out of this place," I told my mom. She told me to go visit my friend Emma in the gym, so I navigated my way down the jam-packed bleachers and into the welcoming cold air of the gym. Minutes later, Emma and I were chatting away. Nothing of importance happened that morning, besides that someone's "breakfast" ended up in the pool, and somehow, a frog jumped into the pool, from who knows where. I mean, where do you get a frog in the middle of winter?! That afternoon, I would be swimming the 100 yard backstroke, 50 yard freestyle, and 50 yard butterfly. I was nervous for my 100 back, because to be able to do a flip turn, you need to know how many strokes from the flags to the wall you have, and at every pool, it is a little bit different. We had talked to the meet officials, as always, and they said that they would use the personal strobe light and hand signals for me since I cannot use my implant while I swim. We always 'remind' them when I register for swim meets that I am deaf and will need someone to use hand signals with me and a parent with me to hold my implant... it doesn't always work the way it should though.

Now I'm next to the block getting really nervous! The official is setting up the strobe light under the blocks for my backstroke event, and I'm handing my implant to my mom. I hop into the 30° below water. The fellow who does hand signals does them wrong and at the wrong time! AYE AYE AYE YA! But that doesn't matter, because I turn to look at my personal strobe light! 1 point for Regan! BUT WAIT, IT DOESN'T GO OFF! I see all of the other swimmers have already started racing! I take off swimming at this point—MAD. 2 points for Regan! Swimming mad must help because I CRUSHED my previous time by *8 seconds*! WOAH! I'm really happy! My time is pretty close to an 11-12 B time, and I only just aged up! My mom wasn't happy with the officials since they didn't start me fairly. She wanted me to call it an unfair start, and re-swim it. I did not want to, because I was more than happy with my time. The other two events went okay that day and I just watched the main strobe light at the pool, rather than the person who did not know how to signal me. I didn't make any new records other than for my 100 backstroke.

Thank goodness we went to the swim meet the next day in the afternoon. I didn't know if I could take another 9 hour swim meet! Today I would be swimming 100 fly, 50 back, and 100 freestyle. I was so worried that in my 100 fly, I would either swim very slowly or be disqualified. I swam my 50 backstroke and YES, the strobe light worked! I beat my old time by 4 seconds! Next, my 100 freestyle. The whole race, I was pushing myself by thinking that I was swimming to save my sister Ryan's life. I came in first in my heat by a LOT! (I did end up saving my sister!). After the race, I could barely get out of the water, and when I did, my legs didn't work. I really gave it my all! Next Race: 100 butterfly. Most people consider butterfly the hardest stroke, and I agree with that, but I think my worst stroke is breaststroke. I had never swam a 100 fly in a meet before. It was such a long distance in a difficult stroke. I was so nervous! I got up onto the block and started when I was signaled. I would soon find out something was horribly wrong- he signaled me wrong and I was the only one racing! At that moment, I knew that it was a false start, but I didn't know what to do, so I just kept swimming hoping that somehow they were timing me. My mom said that the officials were yelling at me and waving their arms for me to stop, the entire crowd watched me at top speed alone in the pool. In the stands my mother was so angry at those people- two days worth of not knowing what they were doing. It's not like this was my first swim meet with these people. On deck, my dad watched as the referee reached in and grabbed me out of the water. It was so embarrassing! That walk back to the other side of the pool was dreadful. Everyone was staring at me, wondering, I am sure, why I just didn't stop when they hollered to me, not knowing that I have a hearing loss. I kept my head held high and returned to the blocks. I swam it again but didn't do well at all! Swimming is hard when you can't hear what is going on. I had had it with those officials!

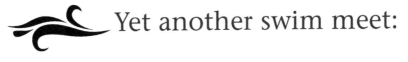 Yet another swim meet:

This swim meet was called the Bronze Championships. It is for people who do not have a B cut time in their age group. This meet was in Akron, which was about 50 minutes away from my house. Thank goodness it was in the afternoon! The night before had been spent at a sleepover at my friend Erin's house, so I was a bit tired and very nervous! This was my last meet of the season so I needed to do GOOD and impress my parents and myself. I thought that the warm-ups started at 1:15 p.m., which is when we got there, but they didn't end up starting until 1:50 p.m., UGHHH! When we arrived, there were people everywhere. There were people coming out of the morning session and coming in for the afternoon session. People were squeezed into corners and there was no room to move. I was trying to figure out how to sign in, where to put my stuff, and trying to figure out if my dad could get a name tag to go on the pool deck with me. Eventually, we got daddy a name tag and we figured out where we could sign in. I looked to see if my friend Isabella had signed in yet. Isabella is an on-again/off-again friend. Some days she's nice to me, others, she's not. She is becoming popular, and doesn't seem to notice me around certain people. When I saw that she hadn't signed in yet, I went to put my stuff on deck. They were still finishing up the morning swim session, but I was GLAD to get settled. I found Isabella, and we hung out until the warm-ups started. She decided to be nice to me that day. Thank goodness! The pool was very big, and I was really psyched, ready to swim my butt off! When it was time for my first event, 50 free, I went to stand in my lane. I asked daddy if I should remind the officials to do hand signals, and he said he would do it instead. I decided to only watch the hand signals to figure out when it was time to "take your mark." I would watch the light for the actual start. I usually swim in the lane second closest to the officials so that I can see them and the strobe light. It also allows me to see the swimmer in the first lane getting up on the starting blocks. For my freestyle, I got a time of 35.something seconds. Thank goodness I got out of the 36 second range, where I had been hanging around for awhile. YES! Next I had my 100 backstroke, which I was really excited about, because the last time I swam it, I was really close to the B time. They used the light under my block to start. I WAS SO READY, JUST LET THE STINKIN' LIGHT GO OFF ALREADY!!! The light went off and I did a perfect start/streamline. Why was everyone waving their arms? I realized that this was another false start. BLEH! I swam back and started over. I swear that it took another five minutes for the light to go off again. When it did, I was already half way down the pool! I had so much adrenaline streaming through me and I was swimming with perfect tempo! I wasn't even tired by my first fifty! I gave every last bit of energy to that last lap, and boy was I just zooming! When I hit that wall, I immediately knew that I had beat my time and I earned a B time at last! I looked up at the scoreboard to see a 1.25:something!!! WOW! My dad was so happy for me, he couldn't stop talking about it! WOW! It was my first B time as an 11 year old! WOW! My coaches all said that it was an amazing swim! WOW! WOW! WOW!

Next my 50 fly! Lately my butterfly had not been improving much. I was hoping to take a lot of time off today. Unfortunately, I again, only improved by a tenth of a second, oh well. Last event: 50 backstroke. My mom drove all of the way down to Akron when she was working to see me swim this event. I was so excited to swim this in front of her! I had to help the official set up the strobe light under my starting block. The official gave me a thumbs up and winked at me. I smiled back. I was so excited to swim for my mom, and impress her and reward her for traveling all of the way down to see me. When the light went off, I did a perfect start, and before I knew it, I was at the other end, and whaddayaknow! I came in first against some twelve year olds with a B time of 39 seconds! WOW! On my 100 back, it is pretty easy to shave off 3 seconds, but on a 50! SO COOL! Next was my freestyle relay. We had to swim against boys, and I had the fastest time on my relay. I was able to gain the lead for us, but our anchor ended up losing the race. I ended up winning 8th place in 100 back against all 11 and 12 year olds that day. We went out to eat that night and didn't get home until 10:00 p.m. I still had homework to do- BLEH. Even so, this was my best swim meet and a great way to end the season!

You may be asking yourself how I wear my implant at these swim meets. When I am just waiting around on the pool deck hanging out, I wear my implant in a little pouch that hangs down around my neck, or I just hold my processor. I am usually covered up with a towel too, since I am always cold. If I am about to swim an event, I hand my processer and pouch to my mom or dad and they hold it while I swim. Hand signals are used for deaf swimmers because we cannot hear the officials calling out directions. Basically, there are three signals that are used: one for taking the 'starting position' either on the blocks or in the water (for backstroke), one for 'take your mark' and one for 'go!' A bright strobe light is also used with the hand signals or the officials voice to start the race.

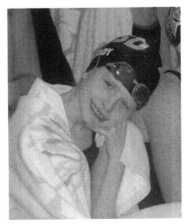

Waiting around at a swim meet.

When I register for a swim meet, my mom emails the meet director to let them know I will be in the meet. We also give them a form we made up that looks like this:

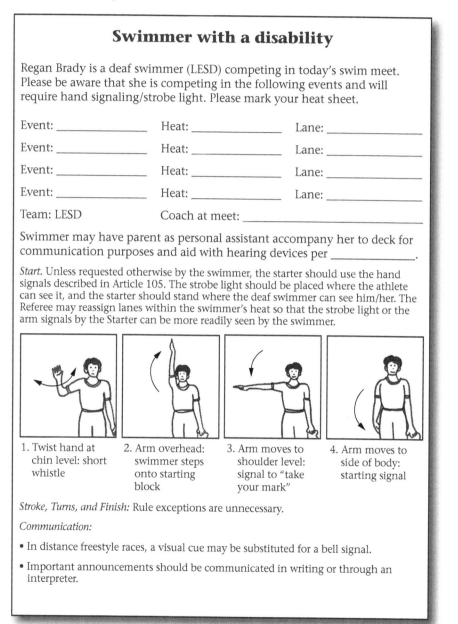

Swimmer with a disability

Regan Brady is a deaf swimmer (LESD) competing in today's swim meet. Please be aware that she is competing in the following events and will require hand signaling/strobe light. Please mark your heat sheet.

Event: _____ Heat: _____ Lane: _____

Event: _____ Heat: _____ Lane: _____

Event: _____ Heat: _____ Lane: _____

Event: _____ Heat: _____ Lane: _____

Team: LESD   Coach at meet: _____

Swimmer may have parent as personal assistant accompany her to deck for communication purposes and aid with hearing devices per _____.

Start. Unless requested otherwise by the swimmer, the starter should use the hand signals described in Article 105. The strobe light should be placed where the athlete can see it, and the starter should stand where the deaf swimmer can see him/her. The Referee may reassign lanes within the swimmer's heat so that the strobe light or the arm signals by the Starter can be more readily seen by the swimmer.

1. Twist hand at chin level: short whistle

2. Arm overhead: swimmer steps onto starting block

3. Arm moves to shoulder level: signal to "take your mark"

4. Arm moves to side of body: starting signal

Stroke, Turns, and Finish: Rule exceptions are unnecessary.

Communication:

• In distance freestyle races, a visual cue may be substituted for a bell signal.

• Important announcements should be communicated in writing or through an interpreter.

Form used with permission from the USA swimming rulebook.

Special Opportunities

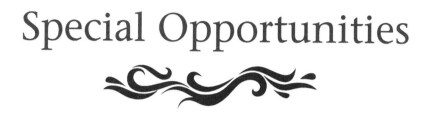

Some people may think that if you have a hearing loss or 'disability', that you are not important or may be overlooked in life. I know that this is completely FALSE! This section will tell you about some of my special opportunities I have had just because of my hearing loss.

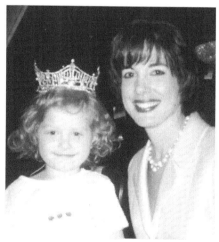

Meeting Heather Whitestone.

Meeting Miss America and Dr. Ling: When I was 4, I had a chance to meet Miss America 1995, Heather Whitestone. I met her at an Auditory-Verbal convention in Baltimore, Maryland. Ms. Whitestone is deaf and was the guest speaker there. Even though we had to wait in a LONG line, it was so exciting to meet such a famous person! I had a chance to wear her crown and have my picture taken with her. My sister and I also have an autographed picture of her.

Since then, I have read a few books about Heather Whitestone. It is so great to see successful people with a hearing loss. I also had a chance to meet Dr. Daniel Ling, one of the founders of AV therapy. Although I was just a baby, I am so glad I have this picture of my family with the late Dr. Ling and his wife.

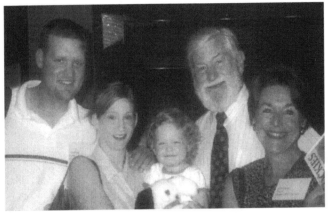

My family with Dr. and Mrs. Daniel Ling.

Being in print:

When I was 6 years old, I was featured on the cover of a magazine called *Advance for Speech-Language Pathologists & Audiologists*. It was a picture of me, Don, and my Mom doing therapy. The magazine did a story on AV therapy and I was mentioned in it. Very cool!

School opportunities:

I really do think that AV has made me a smarter student. I have had many opportunities at school because of my good grades, including participating in Math Olympiad, being named a Great Lakes Scholar, and numerous other school awards. I have also been advanced a few years in math class, which has kept me challenged.

Activities

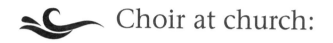

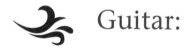 Choir at church:

I have been in my church's choir for two years, beginning in third grade. I enjoy it very much because I love to sing. I am very glad that I am a member of a church choir, because it makes me feel closer to God and it is fun. The truth is, I sing all the time. I drive my family crazy because I am always singing!!

Guitar:

Middle schoolers have the opportunity to take guitar classes. Of course, I chose to do it. I enjoy it a lot, but my fingers get very sore! When I play my guitar with my implant off, I feel like I play so much better. I'm guessing it is because I can hear the song in my head and I can feel the vibrations in my hands. My favorite song to play is "I Hope You Dance" by Lee Ann Womak. I love it and I have a lot of fun playing it.

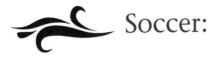 # Soccer:

I play soccer for my city, Shaker Heights. I think that we have one of the best soccer programs around. SYSA (Shaker Youth Soccer Association) has different programs/teams for different skill levels and ages. There is a challenge soccer program, a travel soccer program, and different things beyond that for ultra awesome soccer stars. I play for the challenge team, which is for the good soccer players, but not traveling. My sister plays for the travel team. The challenge team always plays in one spot, which is conveniently located at the end of our street. My dad offered to be the coach for my team, along with another willing dad, so that has been a lot of fun. I recently tried out for and made the U-12 travel soccer team! While I enjoy soccer, and I am a pretty good player, I still believe that water is my natural element.

Crooked River Ensemble:

Crooked River Ensemble is a music and dance group for children in grades 3-7 in the Cleveland area. The ensemble was founded by two teachers at my school, one a dance teacher and the other music (Mrs. Webster). Kids are invited to audition for the ensemble once a year. The first time I auditioned for CRE, I was told I did not make it because they needed to recruit more boys. About half way through the school year, Mrs. Webster contacted my mom asking if I would still like to join CRE. Of course, I said "yes!" What made CRE really fun was that the kids really created the dances and music, rather than just being told what to do. CRE follows a method called Orff Schulwerk. Last year we were invited to perform in Milwaukee at a national convention for music teachers and also at some local events. I was a little worried because our costumes for Milwaukee were white leotards which we were going to splatter paint to match one of our sets. I was having a real hard time finding a white leotard that would not make my BWP stick out horribly. Of all of the choices of costumes, why would they pick a white leotard??? Leotards fit so tightly… and white?? My mom and I spent a lot of time trying different leotards in the stores and ordering them online. I also asked my dance teacher if I could just wear a large white tee shirt like the boys. She said that if I felt comfortable with that, that would be okay- but I thought it would be better to look like the girls even if my processor stuck out. I tried wearing different sports bras and tank tops under the leotard and I tried wearing wraps over the leotard, but nothing worked out very well. I finally decided that if I splatter painted the leotard very carefully, my processor might not be so noticeable. That was the best that I could do. The trip to Milwaukee was a lot of fun and we performed well. No one mentioned that they noticed my processor.

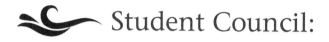 # Student Council:

I just ran for student council representative against two other people in my classroom. I had to give a speech in front of my class, and of course we all had to vote. I WON! I was so happy! Student council meetings are every other Thursday at lunch and recess. Fast forward– I have been to my first seven meetings, and it isn't really as fun as I thought it was going to be. I expected that I would be able to make decisions for the middle school community, but we do a lot of service projects, charity work, and fundraisers. Now don't get me wrong, I'm not saying that this is bad, I just expected different responsibilities!

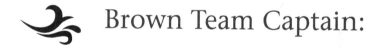 # Brown Team Captain:

My school colors are brown and gold. It is tradition in middle school that you are assigned to either belong to the brown sports team or the gold sports team. I am proud to say that I am on the brown sports team. We have brown and gold days throughout the year in which our teams compete against each other. In the fall we play soccer, in the winter we swim, and in the spring we do track and field. I was excited to be chosen as the brown swim team captain. I think it's a little crazy that I would be chosen as a swim captain. I am a good swimmer, but I can't hear anything while I am in the water! Guess that doesn't matter to anyone!

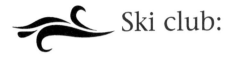 # Ski club:

At my school, once you are in middle school, you are eligible to join ski club. I had been skiing only once in my life, and really enjoyed it, so of course, I begged my parents to let me join. They were somewhat worried about me skiing without them, as they worry about anything that could cause a head injury or make me loose my BTE! We all agreed that if I would wear a ski helmet and agreed to be very careful, I could give ski club a try. I ended up joining and getting one of the last remaining spots!

Buying a helmet that would fit properly with my implant was a bit of a challenge, but it was not as bad as I thought. It was actually easier than finding a bike helmet that fit well because the ski helmets had soft Velcro straps inside that I could adjust to fit around my headpiece well. Maybe I should have worn a ski helmet bike riding all these years.

That Thursday after school, as the bell rang from my last class, I was so excited! I raced back to my locker to grab my things and start changing into my ski clothes. This was the worst part of ski club, everyone crowded around their lockers changing, packing their backpacks and getting their gear. Eventually, I made it to the bus and took off for the slopes. You are probably wondering what slopes are in Cleveland, Ohio. Actually, there are three ski areas in Cleveland, two of them thanks to the Cuyahoga Valley National Park. That is where we were headed, 40 minutes down the road to Boston Mills. We arrived at Boston Mills, rented our skis and ski boots, and put on our helmets, goggles, coats, and gloves. My ski buddy was Cara, a friend, who was a beginner like me. Cara and I soon had our skis on and went outside for our lessons. We didn't have to wait long however, because the instructor soon had us walking around in our skis. After we passed that stage of the lesson, we were taken to the 'bunny hill'. That 'bunny hill' looked quite large to me. Here I learned to bounce on my skis as I went down the slope. I also learned something called pizza and french fries. This is where you make your way down the hill, yelling out pizza (skiing with your tips pointed together) or french fries (skiing with your skis parallel).

After I passed that, I worked on my turns. The last part of my lesson that day was weaving between cones. That was pretty easy, and I completed it quickly. I had completed my lesson and earned my first ski sticker. I was now able to ski on a REAL hill!

The very first time that I went down the 'real' hill, I had a panic attack. I had no control over myself and I didn't stay between the markers on the hill at all! I became better after that and remained in control of things. After about 3 more times down that slope, my friends and I were stopped by an instructor who said that if we went down one more time, and he liked the way that we skied, he would give us a sticker for that hill. So we went down one more time, and got our second sticker for that night! The instructor asked us if we wanted to take the chair lifts to the higher part of the hill. Cara and I were so excited because we had never been on a chair lift before and we wanted to go to the REAL top of the REAL hill! We were shown how to get on and off of the chair lifts and in only a few peaceful minutes, we were at the peak. Wow, the hill looked so big from the top! I was nervous but used what I had learned to control my speed that first time down. It was so fun! At that moment knew that I was hooked! Cara felt the same as me, and we became ski buddies. Even though this was only my second time skiing, I knew that I was hooked for life. Soon as it was 7:30 p.m., and time already to change, put our skis away, and get on the bus for the ride back to school.

My hearing loss didn't get in the way of skiing. I did learn that wearing the longest possible cord with my BWP helped. With all the extra clothes pulling on me, the extra length helped keep my headpiece from falling off. I only wore my BWP because I was afraid of my BTE falling off. Of course, I kept an extra battery zipped in my pocket. I also remembered to sit on the left of Cara as we rode the chairlifts so I could hear her better with my right side. I think the biggest problem for a hearing impaired skier would be finding a helmet that fit well with hearing aids or implants.

Music

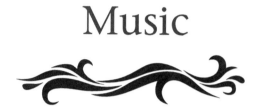

My iPod is a silver nano. I listen to my iPod A LOT more now because of something that I learned I can do. I learned that by using a cable, I could connect my iPod directly to my BWP and listen to music using a 50/50 sound ratio. What I mean is that my microphone is configured so that I can hear 50% of regular noise and 50% of what I am connected to. For Christmas, I received this cable along with a big binder of lyrics that my parents created of new songs they put on my iPod. The lyrics are very helpful to me because, as you know, music can be hard for even hearing people to decipher sometimes. The lyrics allow me to follow along with songs and learn the words. I was so grateful for that gift. I was soon listening to my iPod more than ever with this new method. Later, that same day, I found an audio jack in my dad's car that looked interesting. I cautiously plugged one end of my new cable into it and the other into my processor. I was soon listening to the DVD's in the car this way! This was all accomplished using a cable that you can find at your local Target store or RadioShack. I hope that this is helpful for all you BWP-wearing-music-lovers. I can also plug directly into my BTE, which I sometimes do to practice listening with just that ear.

Interviews

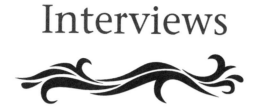

I interviewed a few people to see how they viewed my hearing loss.

 ## Interview with my sister Ryan who is 7

Q: *So, Ryan, you know that you sister, Regan is deaf, how does that make you feel?*
A: It doesn't make a big difference to me.

Q: *How does it impact your life?*
A: Sometimes it is a little harder for me like at swimming when people forget that you are deaf and try and talk to you. I have to kind of, like tell you what they are saying in a different way.

Q: *What are some other ways that it affects your life?*
A: When we sleep together at night, I try and talk to you because I don't know if you have your sound on or not.

Q: *Do any of your friends know about my hearing loss?*
A: One of them.

Q: *Does she ever say anything to you about it?*
A: She asked, "What is that thing on your sister's ear?"

Q: *How did you respond?*
A: "Well she's deaf and that is to help her hear. Don't tell anybody."

Q: **Why did you say, "Don't tell anybody?"**
A: I don't know. Because I didn't think that you wanted her to know.

Q: *What do you want to be when you grow up?*
A: An archeologist.

Q: *Why do you want to be one?*
A: Cause I want to find cool stuff in the ground.

Q: *What is your biggest hope or dream?*
A: That people stop polluting and littering.

Q: *Who is your best role model?*
A: Either you or Esme, our neighbor.

Q: *What are the qualities they have that make you want to be like them?*
A: Because they are funny, nice, friendly, and cool.

C: *Thank you for letting me interview you Ryan!*
A: You're welcome!

 # Thoughts from my music teacher, Mrs. Webster

Mrs. Webster has been my music teacher since first grade. She also runs Crooked River Ensemble and my church's youth choir. Mrs. Webster first learned that I was deaf when she met with my parents and other teachers before first grade to talk about my needs. This however, was before she met me in person. Mrs. Webster said she thought that a deaf student would not be able to learn music. She also thought that she would have to change the whole class curriculum and teaching style so that I could learn. She said that she thought that the hardest part of teaching a deaf person music would be teaching pitch. She worried that my pitch would be far off and I would sound very wrong. Mrs. Webster's mother had hearing loss in one ear, and Mrs. Webster actually remembers taking sign language classes with her mother when she was a young girl. Mrs. Webster told me that she was amazed when I walked in and I could talk fine, and I had perfect pitch. She said that she would often tell people how I was even beyond "normal" when I could sing better than even the normally hearing kids!

⌇ Interview with my 4th grade teacher Ms. Boutton:

Q: *Did you know, before I reached 4th grade that there was hearing impaired student in school?*

A: Yes, I knew that there was a student with a hearing loss because I chatted with you and your mother informally when you first came to HB because we were fellow West Siders. I talked to your mom and you a few times before I ever knew that you had a hearing loss. I think I actually found out about your hearing from another teacher.

Q: *What were your initial thoughts about me? Any preconceived ideas?*

A: Well, my initial thoughts about you were that you were very cute, very well mannered, and intelligent. You also were always smiling so I thought you were a very happy child. I didn't have preconceived ideas because I formed my initial thoughts about you before I was aware that you had a hearing loss. Finding that out didn't change anything. You were still Regan.

Q: *How was I the same/different from what you originally imagined?*

A: When you became my student, my original impressions about you held true. You were indeed well mannered, intelligent, cheerful, and very cute (but in a more mature way, of course). I respected you a great deal because you were your own advocate, you didn't try to get extra attention or make excuses for yourself, and you handled your situation very matter-of-factly. You also blew me away with your math thinking--I was ready to turn the class over to you on more than one occasion.

Q: *Was it difficult for you to have me in the classroom?*

A: No, it was not difficult to have you in the classroom. In fact, it was fascinating. I loved learning about your implant, how it worked, and how to help you out if you needed it (which you rarely did). It was very interesting to talk to your AV therapist and read the materials he gave me. You were very self-sufficient and most of the time I didn't really need think too much about it. I loved using the microphone because it helped everyone pay attention and hear what I was saying, and I didn't have to talk loudly all day. So any adaptive measures we had to take benefited the entire class, and did not make things more difficult. The only time I was concerned was at Shaker Village at night; I wanted to make sure that the adults knew to look out for you in case of an emergency. I also watched your speech and writing a little more closely to make sure that your skills were developing appropriately because I have a very good friend who's daughter has a hearing loss and knew from talking to her that language development could sometimes be a problem. Most of the time I just enjoyed you because you were you, and you were (and still are) a great girl who was fun to be around. The hearing was just a small piece of you. Every student presents her own special set of needs and talents; that's the fun part about being a teacher!

My Poetry

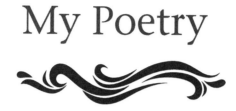

Chili
BY REGAN BRADY 3RD GRADE

I see
the steam evaporating
into
nothingness
from the pot
swirling,
a race to the ceiling
I hear
the rhythmic chopping
of the vegetables
and the 'plop' into the pot
I smell
the freshness
of the carrots
and the smell of
halfway-done homemade chili
I feel
the stubbornness of the meat
as I stir
I feel the dampness on my face
when the water vapor
kisses it
as I lean over the pot
I taste the spicy completed chili
made from hand-
tastes so good

Eraser

BY REGAN BRADY 4TH GRADE

Sitting
Waiting

For someone to make
a mistake

Slowly,
as my user
becomes more
careless

I start to
wear away

My pink
rubbery skin
begins to turn black

But I know my deeds
free the world
from
mistakes

MUD

BY REGAN BRADY 5TH GRADE

Mud is a stain
A concoction of rain and soil
On my white clothes
And imperfection on my ego
Worms call for help
Drowning in the mass
Of oozy slime
The single fault
On the shiny linoleum floor
A stain on my Sunday best
A splat on my pale shirt
Mud baked pies on my driveway
Though my mother doesn't find them
as delightful as I do-
Mud
Mud
Mud
A big brown blemish

My thoughts on technology

I have mixed feelings when I take a step into the real world. Full of beeping, buzzing, music, radio, and T.V. I see people texting and driving, yakking on phones while waiting in line at the bank. Technology: Good or bad? I say both. Technology is very important to many people, because their jobs, fortune, and well, life depend on it. It is especially important to all of the people in the medical field, because without technology, we wouldn't have all of the fancy tools, machines, and medicines needed to stay healthy. I have a direct connection to this, because my implants are pure technology. Without them, I cannot hear. To a certain extent technology is amazing, but when applications (games) for phones, computers, etc. replace normal everyday utilities, it becomes too much. There are now electronic books and apps for finding your cell phone or your loved one. When this starts to happen, I believe that the human race is depending on technology too much. I start to wonder if we would be better off without all of these "new-fangled" devices. Maybe kids should go out and play instead of being cooped up in their room all day playing video games. So, to answer my own question, is technology good or bad, I would definitely answer that it is good, in moderation.

I hope that over time, as technology advances, implant processors will improve and become smaller. Smaller and thinner would be good, and maybe even completely internal! I would love if the amazing scientists of the 21st century could perhaps enhance the sound as much to be at the level of hearing people! With the knowledge of people these days, the "impossible" is constantly changing!

So, there you have it, my life's story in 60 some pages! What I want people to walk away knowing is that I love to hear, I love my implants, and anything is possible—DREAM BIG!!!

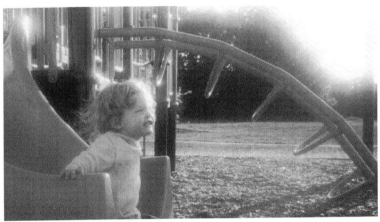

Regan dreaming big!

Swimmer with a disability*

_____ is a deaf swimmer competing in today's swim meet. Please be aware that she is competing in the following events and will require hand signaling/strobe light. Please mark your heat sheet.

Event: _____   Heat: _____   Lane: _____

Event: _____   Heat: _____   Lane: _____

Event: _____   Heat: _____   Lane: _____

Event: _____   Heat: _____   Lane: _____

Team: _____   Coach at meet: _____

Swimmer may have parent as personal assistant accompany her to deck for communication purposes and aid with hearing devices per _____.

Start. Unless requested otherwise by the swimmer, the starter should use the hand signals described in Article 105. The strobe light should be placed where the athlete can see it, and the starter should stand where the deaf swimmer can see him/her. The Referee may reassign lanes within the swimmer's heat so that the strobe light or the arm signals by the Starter can be more readily seen by the swimmer.

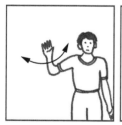 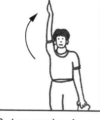 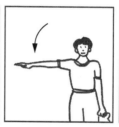 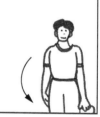

1. Twist hand at chin level: short whistle

2. Arm overhead: swimmer steps onto starting block

3. Arm moves to shoulder level: signal to "take your mark"

4. Arm moves to side of body: starting signal

Stroke, Turns, and Finish: Rule exceptions are unnecessary.

Communication:

• In distance freestyle races, a visual cue may be substituted for a bell signal.

• Important announcements should be communicated in writing or through an interpreter.

This page may be reproduced without permission

8394125R0

Made in the USA
Charleston, SC
05 June 2011